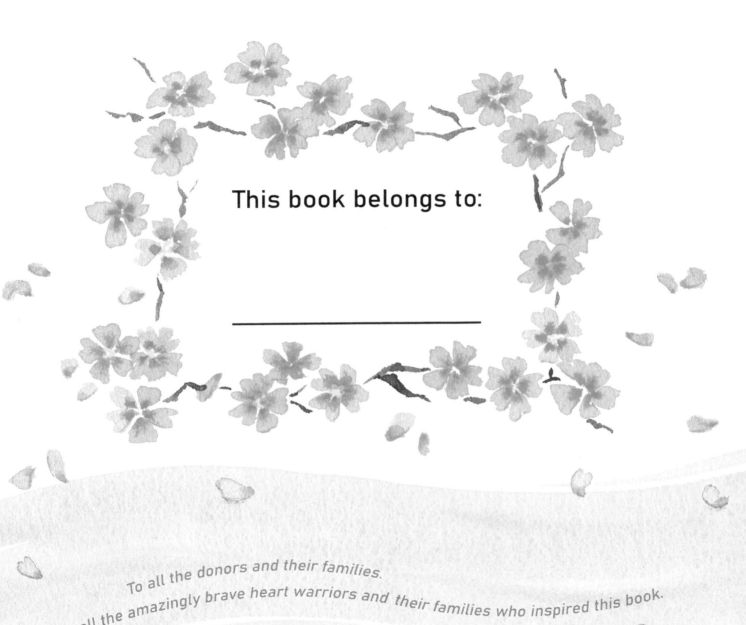

This book belongs to:

_____

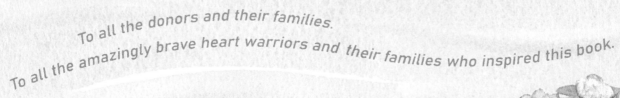

To all the donors and their families.

To all the amazingly brave heart warriors and their families who inspired this book.

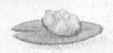
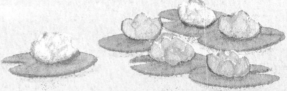

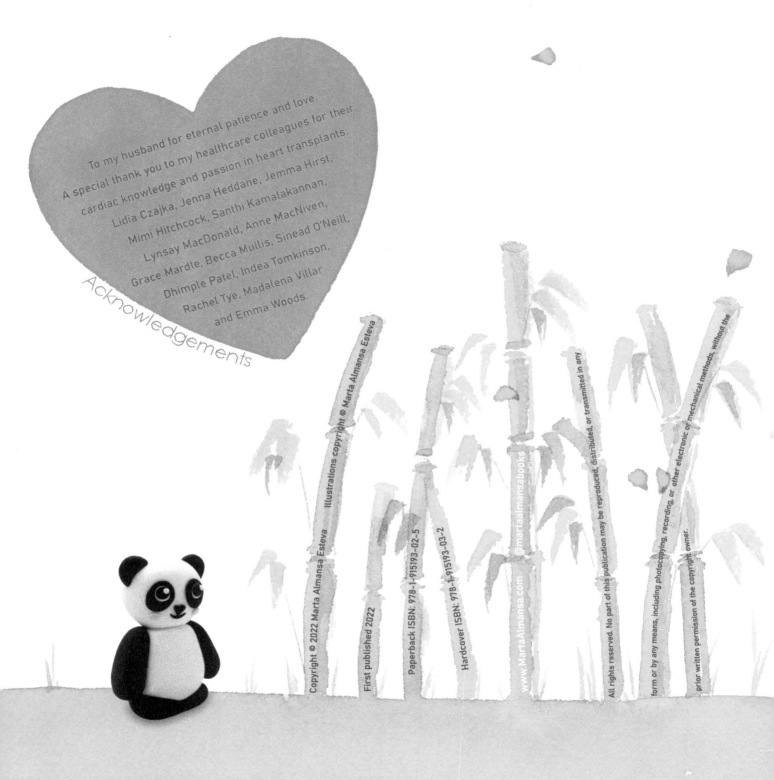

Acknowledgements

To my husband for eternal patience and love.
A special thank you to my healthcare colleagues for their
cardiac knowledge and passion in heart transplants:
Lidia Czajka, Jenna Heddane, Jemma Hirst,
Mimi Hitchcock, Santhi Kamalakannan,
Lynsay MacDonald, Anne MacNiven,
Grace Mardle, Becca Mullis, Sinead O'Neill,
Dhimple Patel, Indea Tomkinson,
Rachel Tye, Madalena Villar
and Emma Woods.

Copyright © 2022 Marta Almansa Esteva

Illustrations copyright © Marta Almansa Esteva

First published 2022

Paperback ISBN: 978-1-915193-02-5

Hardcover ISBN: 978-1-915193-03-2

www.MartaAlmansa.com   @martaalmansabooks

Marta Almansa Esteva

Little panda and her super heart

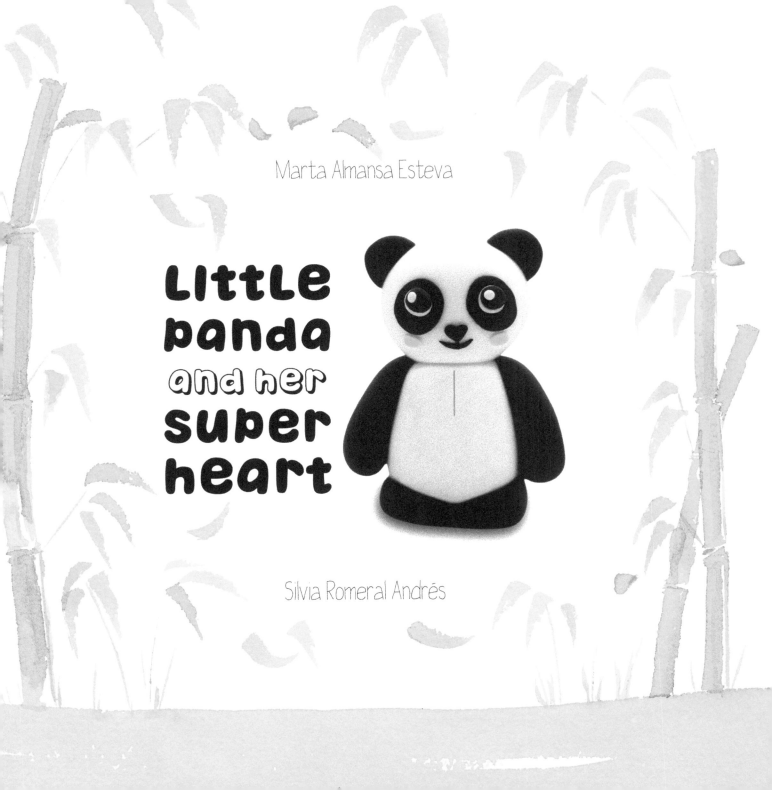

Silvia Romeral Andrés

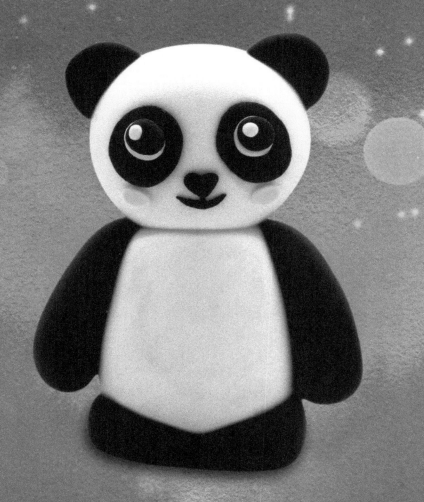

This is Little Panda.
She has a very important secret.

Little Panda knows she is a superhero.
She does not know where her superpowers are.
They might be hiding or taking a nap. All she knows is that
she has to find out where they are, no matter what!

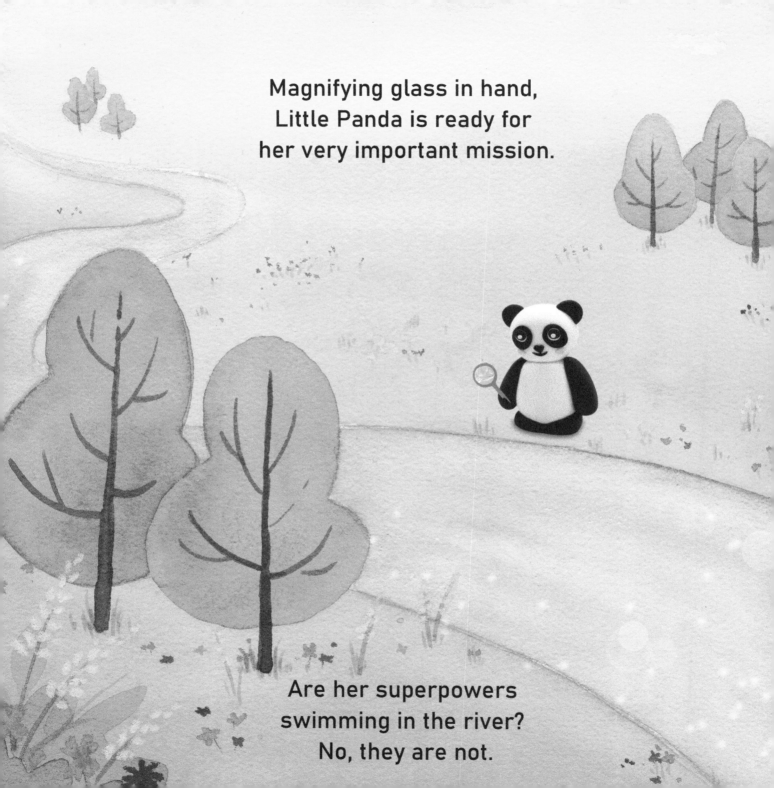

Magnifying glass in hand,
Little Panda is ready for
her very important mission.

Are her superpowers
swimming in the river?
No, they are not.

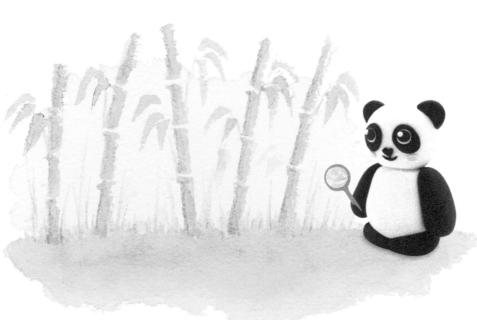

Are they hiding in
a bamboo forest?
They are not,
but this is delicious!

What about inside
the trunk of a tree?
Not there!

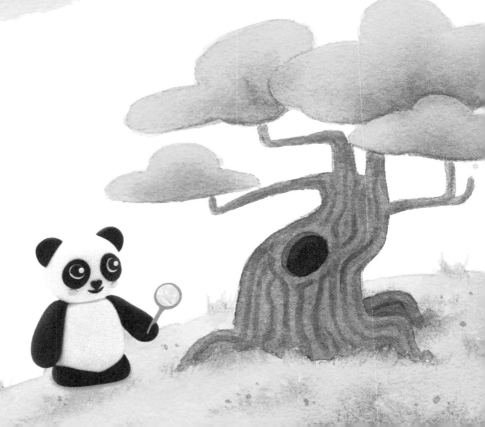

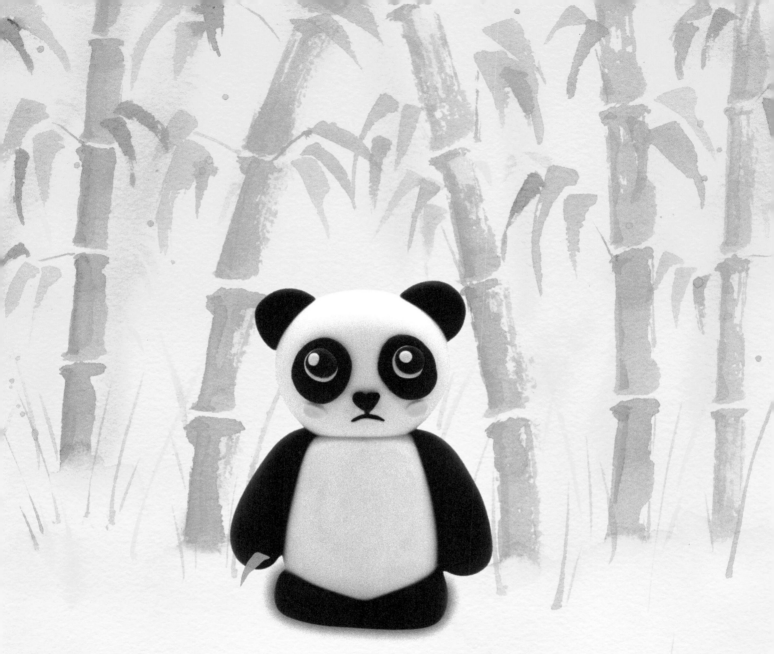

Some days, Little Panda feels weak and does not want to eat.
She does not even want a teeny, tiny bamboo leaf.

"What about fish?" asks Blue Bird.
"No, thanks," says Little Panda.
"Or a pumpkin?" Blue Bird says.
"I'm not hungry," Little Panda replies.

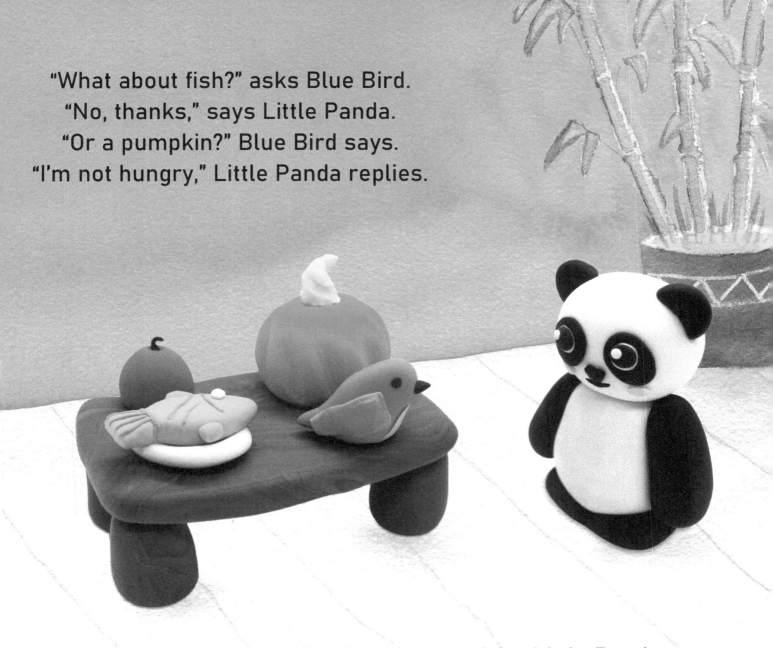

This is not normal for Little Panda.
She is usually full of bamboo and beans!
Something must be wrong.

Today, Little Panda is more tired than usual.
She feels a bit weak, too.
Daddy Panda decides to take
her to the hospital.

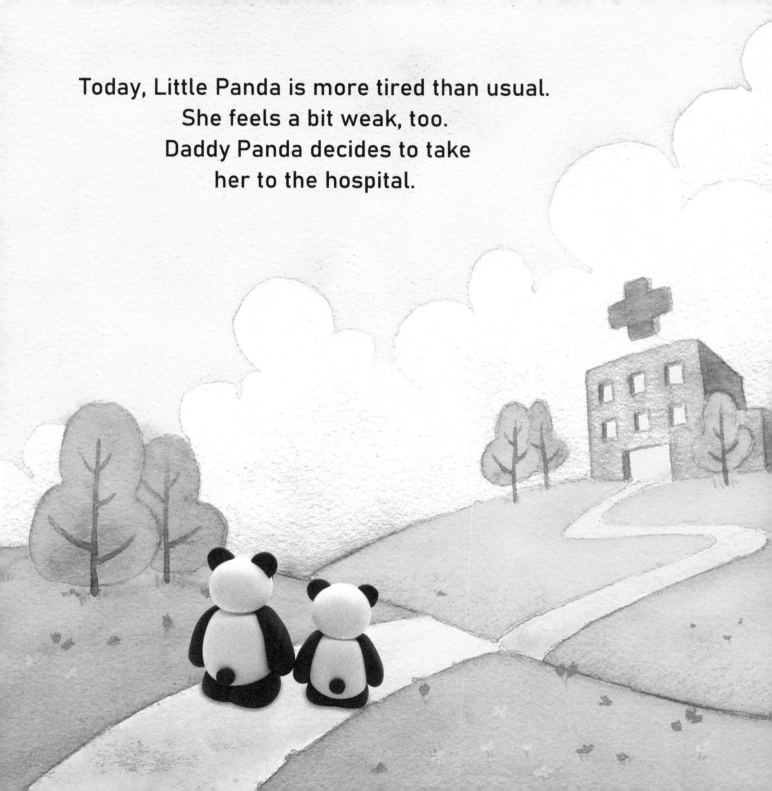

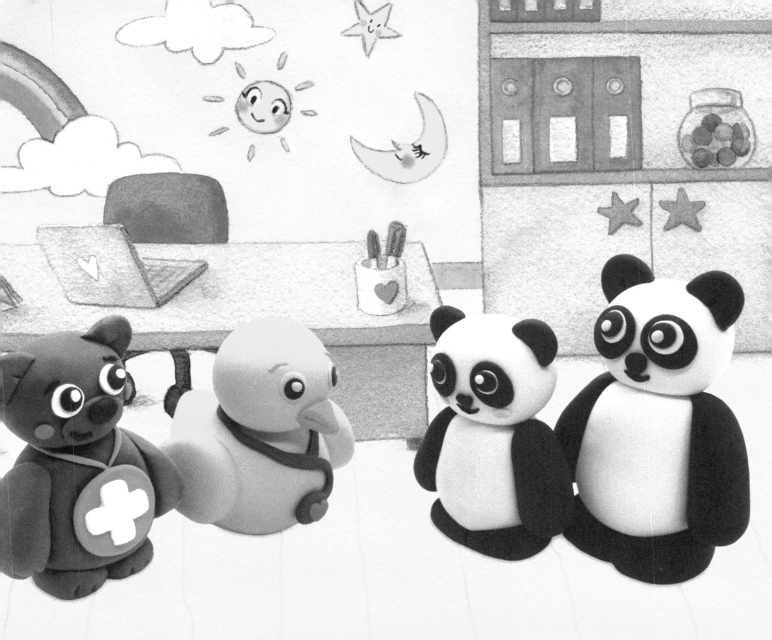

Doctor Duck and Nurse Bear are ready to help them.
They have to do some checks to find out how to help.

The blood pressure monitor tells them how strong Little Panda's heart is.

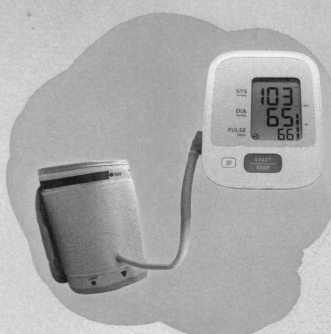

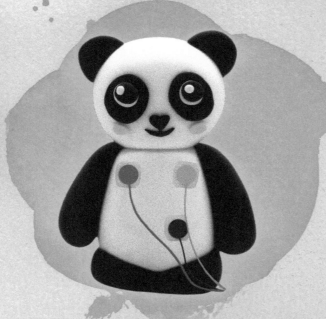

The three ECG stickers look like traffic lights. They show the rhythm of Little Panda's heart.

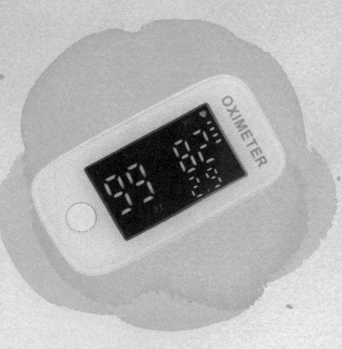

This magic red light
is the pulse oximeter.
It shows how well
Little Panda is breathing.

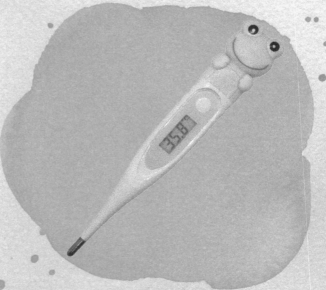

The frog thermometer
shows if she is
too hot or too cold.

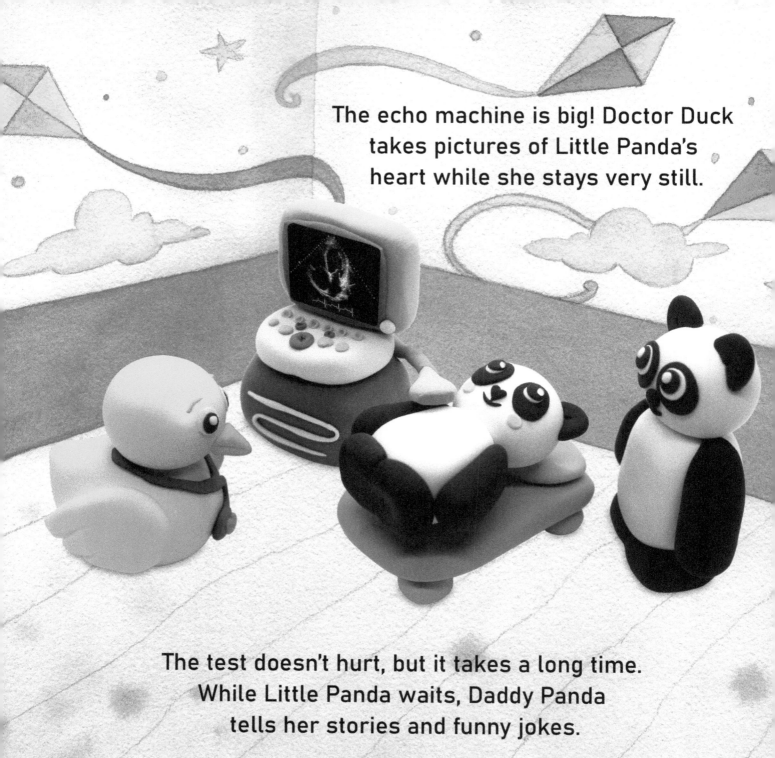

The echo machine is big! Doctor Duck takes pictures of Little Panda's heart while she stays very still.

The test doesn't hurt, but it takes a long time. While Little Panda waits, Daddy Panda tells her stories and funny jokes.

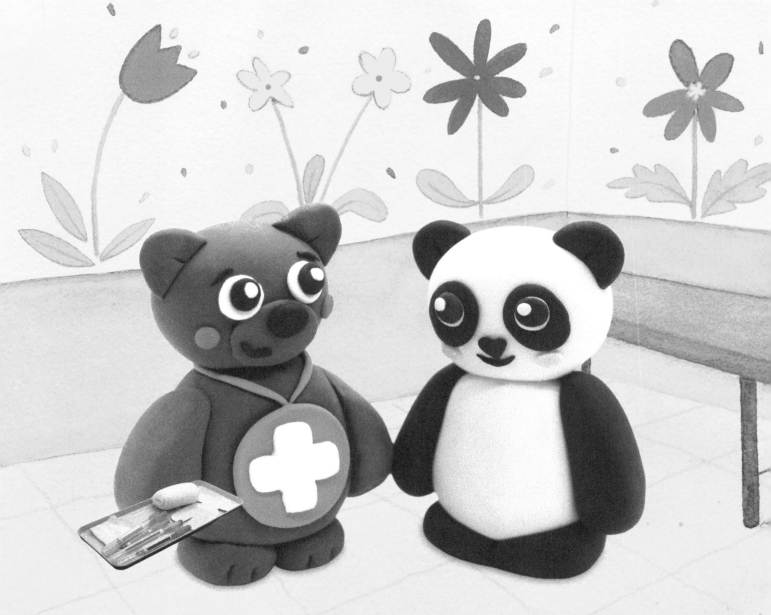

"You have been super brave so far, Little Panda!
We are very proud of you. The last check is a blood test,"
says Nurse Bear. "I'll sing some songs for you.
Which song is your favourite?"

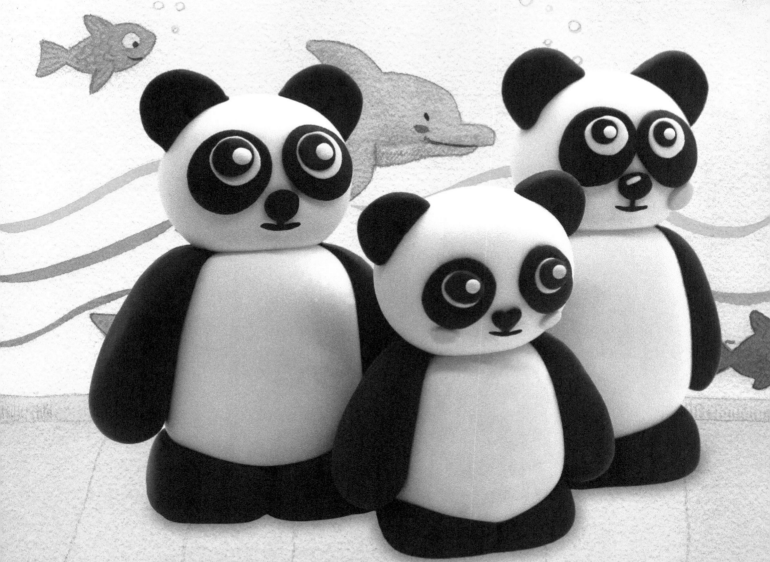

Little Panda has been the bravest panda in town!
When her blood tests are done, the doctors know what's going on.
They know why she does not want even the tastiest bamboo
and why she sometimes feels too tired to climb trees.

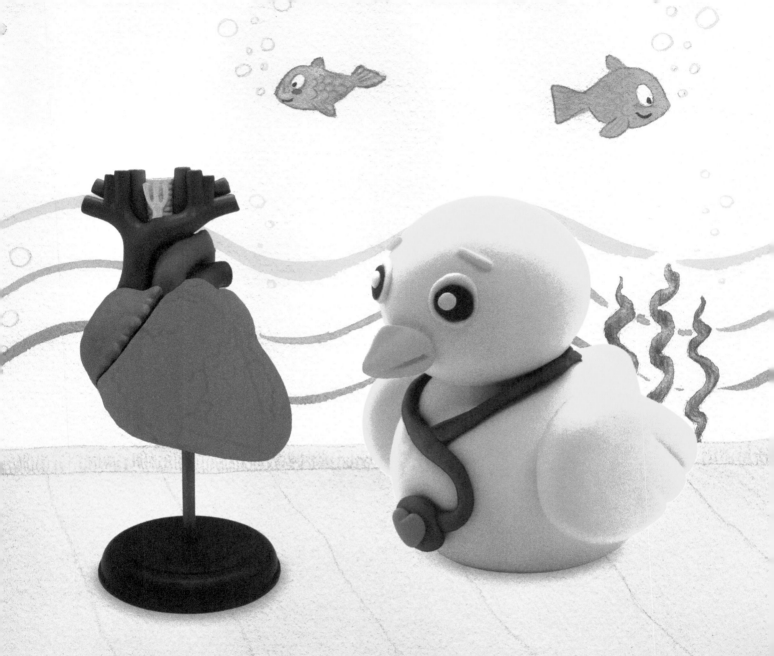

Little Panda's heart is sick. She needs a new heart.
She will wait in the hospital until the new heart arrives.
Mummy and Daddy will be there with her.

There is a big team looking after Little Panda in the hospital to help her feel better while she waits! There are...

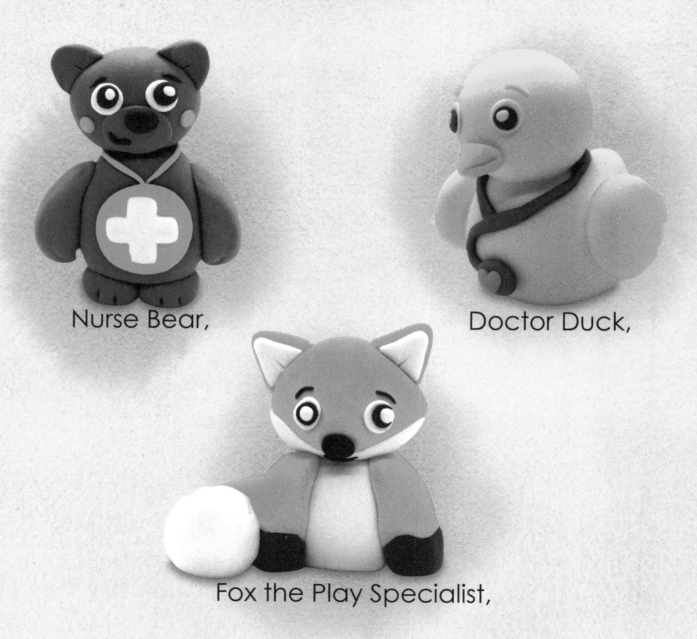

Nurse Bear,

Doctor Duck,

Fox the Play Specialist,

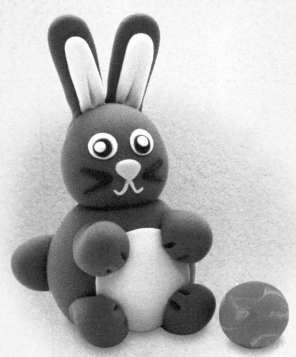

Bunny the Physiotherapist,

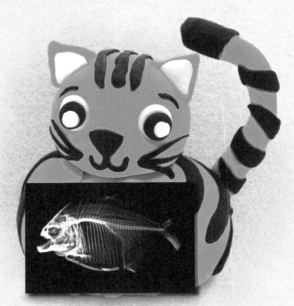

Tiger the Radiographer,

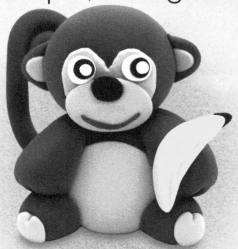

and Monkey the Dietitian.

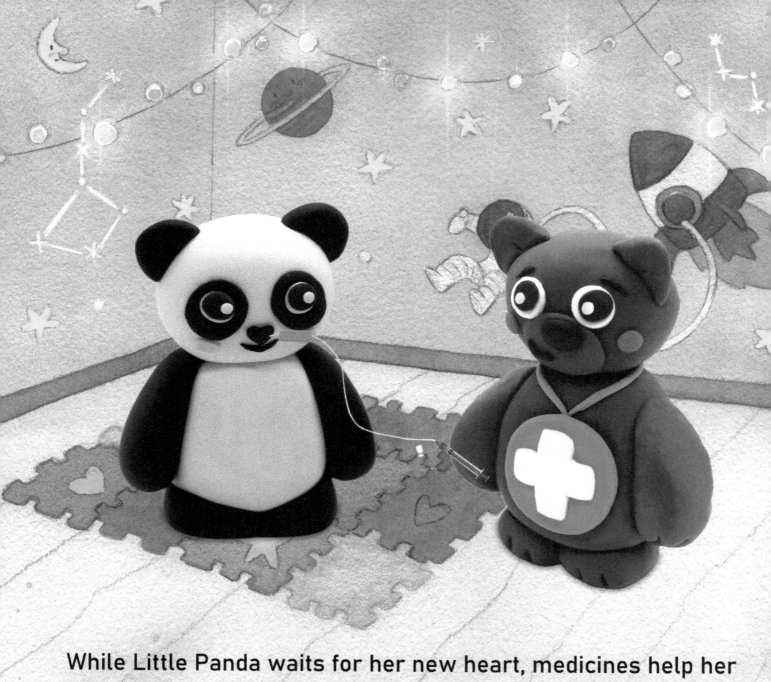

While Little Panda waits for her new heart, medicines help her to feel better. Sometimes, she needs a nasogastric tube so she can have a full tummy even if she does not feel hungry.

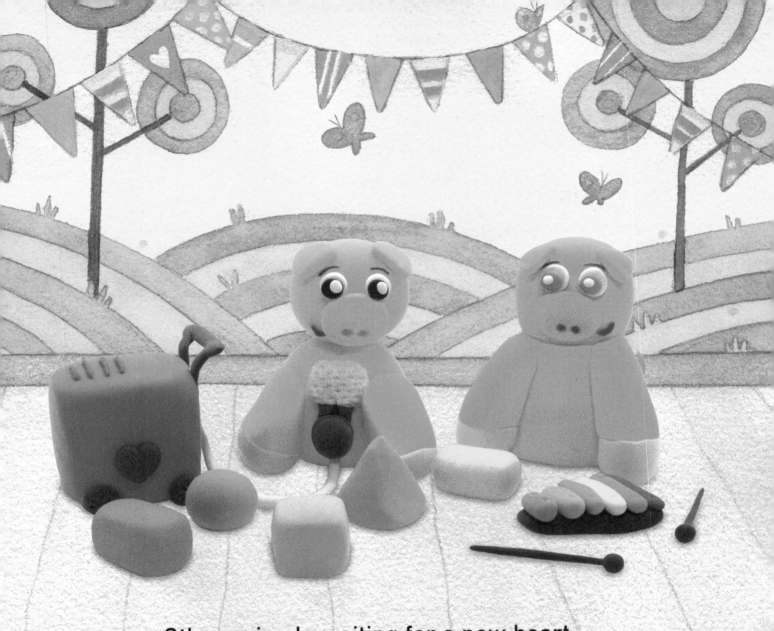

Other animals waiting for a new heart
sometimes need a bit of extra strength.
Doctor Duck connects a great machine to their hearts.
It helps their hearts pump blood around their bodies.

Little Panda waits and waits and waits
for her new heart to arrive.
Some days go fast and are busy!
Some days are slow and tiring.

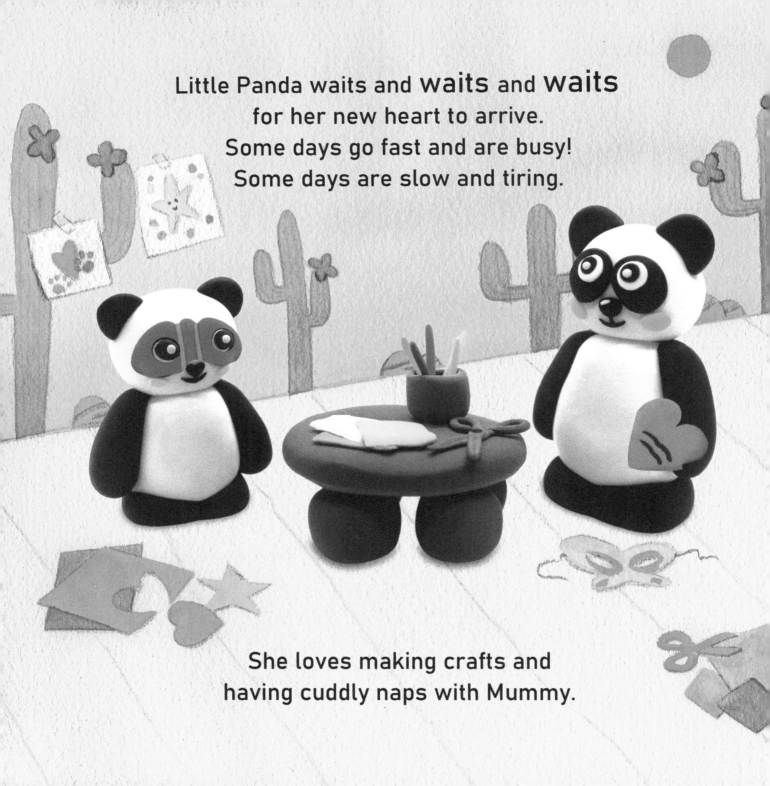

She loves making crafts and
having cuddly naps with Mummy.

She loves colouring with Daddy and
playing instruments with the play specialist.

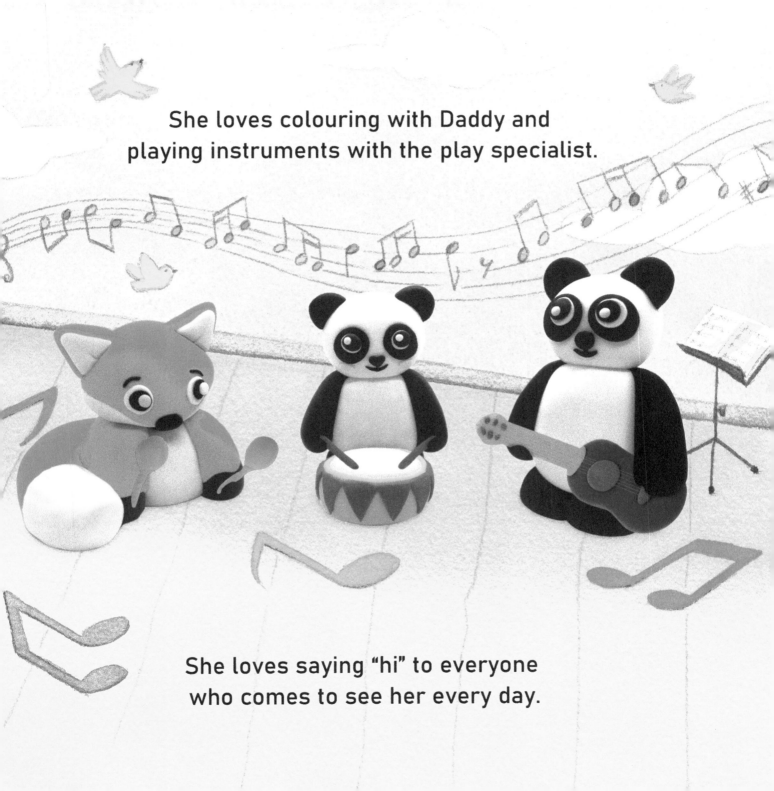

She loves saying "hi" to everyone
who comes to see her every day.

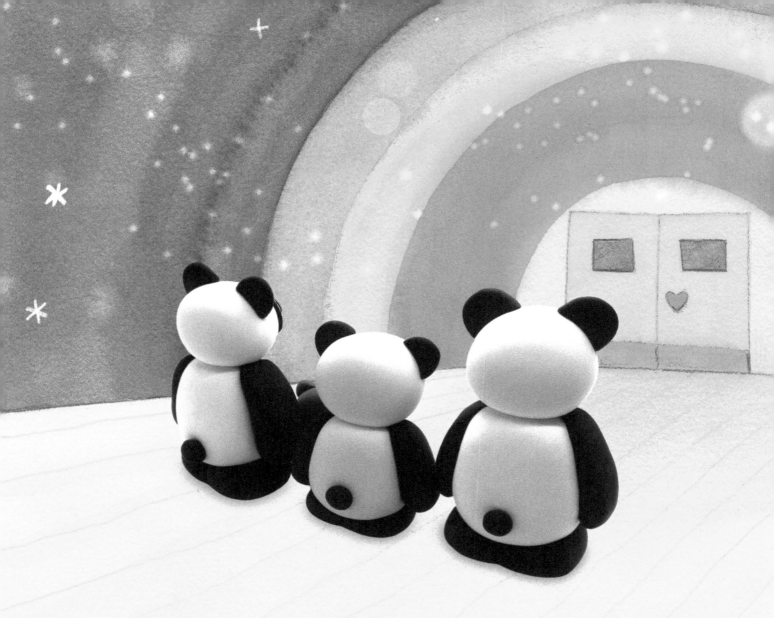

Finally, they get the call!
Little Panda's new heart is ready and waiting for her.
She grabs her teddy and holds her Mummy and Daddy's
hands as they go to theatre together.

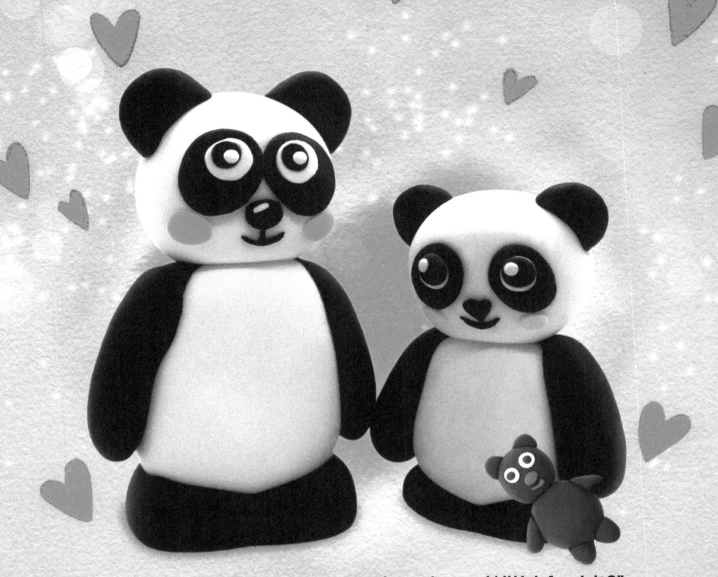

"I am worried. I don't want it to hurt. Will I feel it?"
"No, Little Panda. It won't hurt. They will give you a special
sleepy medicine so you are asleep during the operation.
You won't feel any pain. When it is finished,
Mummy and Daddy will give you a big cuddle."

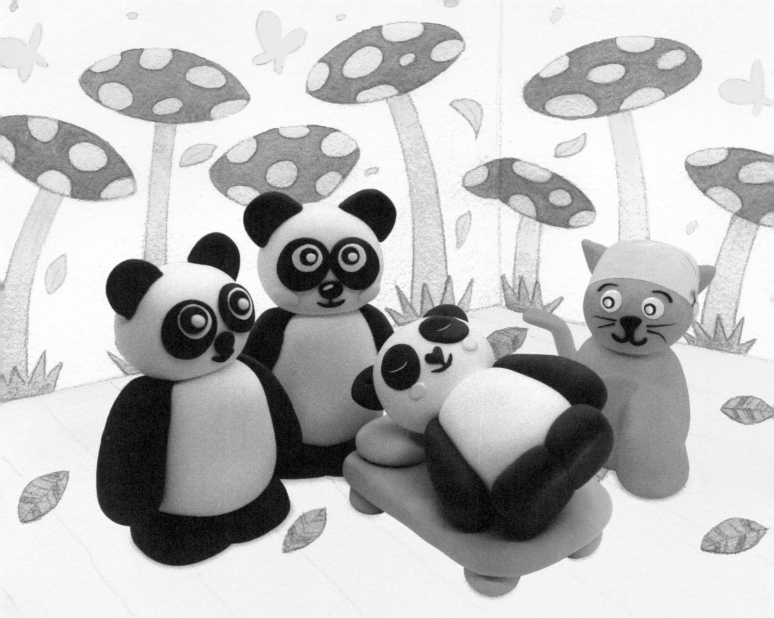

With a kind smile, Cat the Anaesthetist gives Little Panda
her special medicine. Little Panda falls asleep.
While Little Panda's eyes close, Mummy whispers in her ear,
"When you wake up, we'll be right here!"

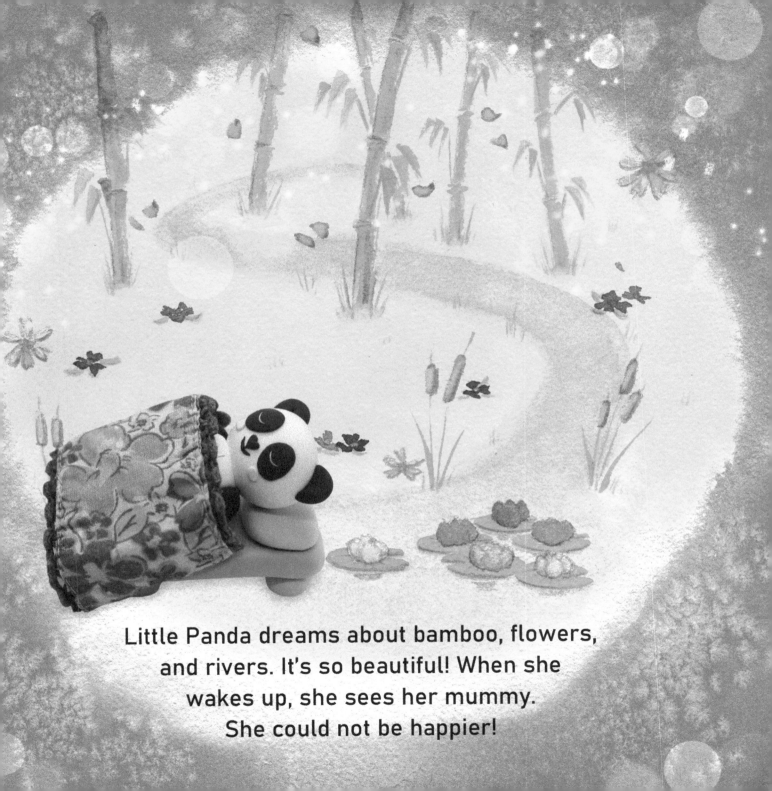

Little Panda dreams about bamboo, flowers,
and rivers. It's so beautiful! When she
wakes up, she sees her mummy.
She could not be happier!

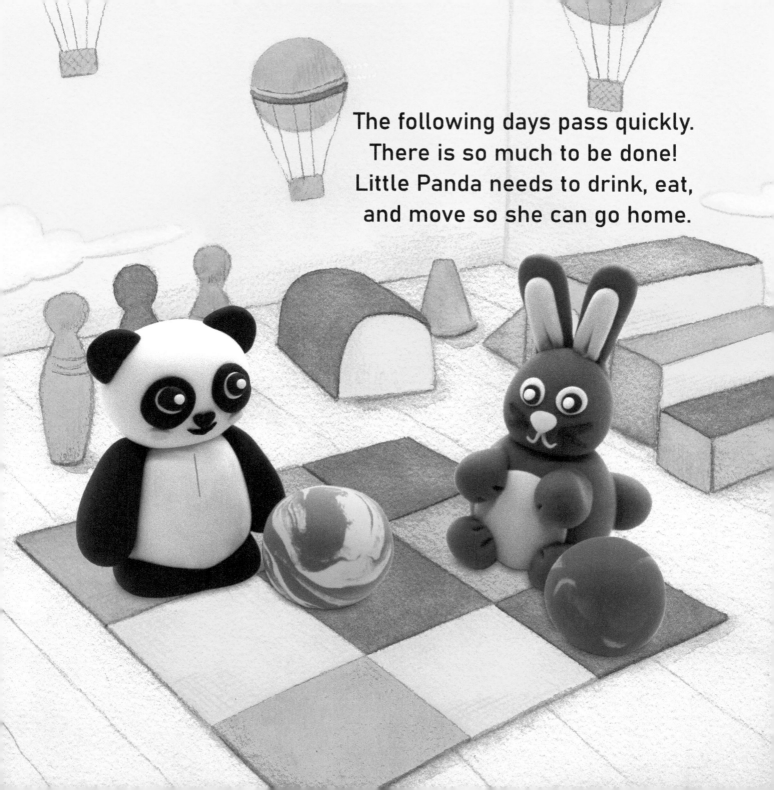

The following days pass quickly.
There is so much to be done!
Little Panda needs to drink, eat,
and move so she can go home.

Little Panda feels different. She feels strong.
She looks at the scar on her chest and
feels proud of herself for being brave.
After all that time in bed, it's nice to be
able to chase the birds!

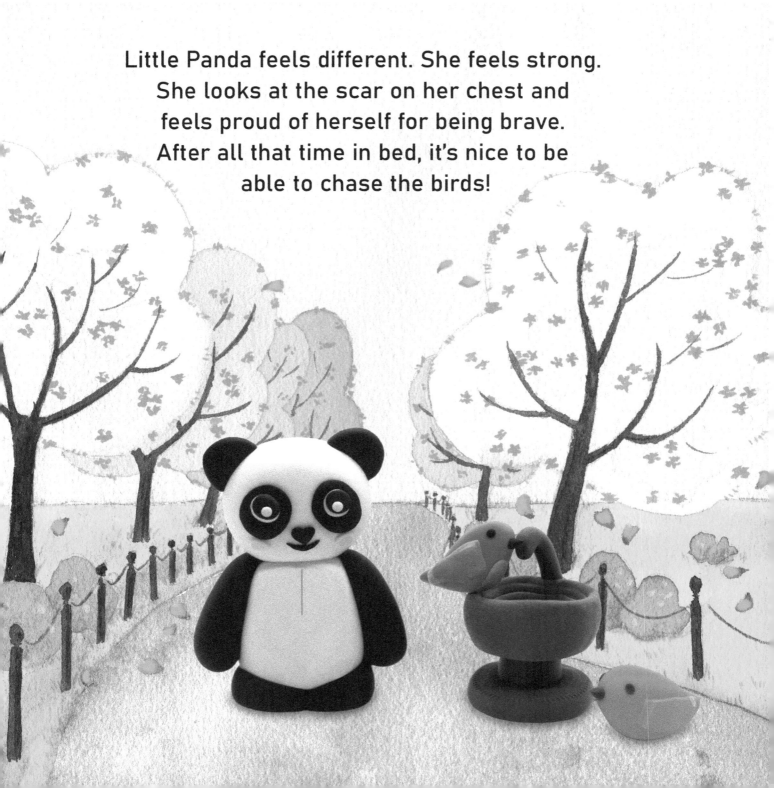

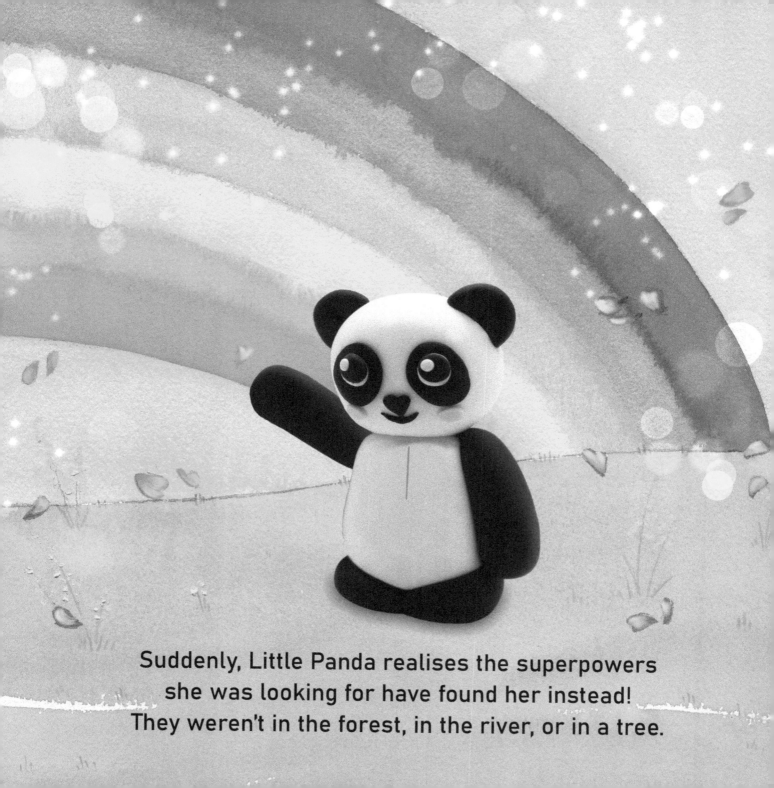

Suddenly, Little Panda realises the superpowers
she was looking for have found her instead!
They weren't in the forest, in the river, or in a tree.

"They are here, inside me!"
Little Panda is a super panda.
Her new heart is her superpower.
It is a super heart!

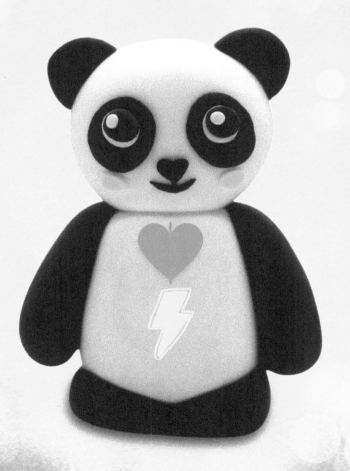

Printed in the USA
CPSIA information can be obtained
at www.ICGtesting.com
LVHW060746260124
769968LV00005B/79